Hearing Aids

101

A Layman's Guide

Thomas Shaw

Hearing Aids 101: A Layman's Guide

By Thomas R Shaw

Disclaimer and FTC Notice

Table of Contents

Why I Wrote This Book

There are many books about hearing aids on the market. Many are highly technical and not really appropriate for the average hearing impaired person. Some are simply a way to try to sell one brand over another.

This book is different from those in many ways. First, it's designed for the person who thinks they have hearing loss and are just starting to explore their options. Second, it's written so that anyone can easily understand it—it is not designed to be a college textbook. Third, it is written by someone who has had almost 20 years of experience helping hearing impaired individuals.

I wrote this book because I know people with hearing loss start out searching for information in order to make the right decision for them. No two hearing losses are the same. And no two individuals are affected by a hearing loss in exactly the same way. If you know, or simply suspect, that you have hearing loss, and that loss is causing you difficulty in your everyday life, then this short book will be a great help to you.

If you find it useful, I would sincerely appreciate a brief review on Amazon. This is the second book I have written, on subjects that I am truly passionate about. The other, Woodworking Shop 101 - How To Set Up A Shop On A Budget, is also available on Amazon for both Kindle and in hard copy.
http://www.amazon.com/dp/B00IXME6HK

My Industry Background

I began my almost 20 year career in this industry at the age of 52 in Phoenix, AZ, dispensing hearing aids 'in-home' in the Valley of the Sun. I was taught by one of the best trainers in the industry and normally performed up to 4 hearing evaluations a day, five days a week. Anyone who has ever sold anything in-home knows that you see a broad cross section of individuals and learn a great deal about life in general. My personal experience certainly attests to that.

Most of my clients were senior citizens. Some were quite elderly, the oldest being just under 100; the youngest was barely 20. They all had one thing in common, they did not hear as well as they used to or wanted to. All of them were seeking information about hearing aids. Some had tried hearing aids without success in the past; others knew almost nothing about hearing aids. All had questions. I often learned as much from them as they learned from me. I do know that I did improve the quality of life for many.

From there I went to Denver, CO, where I helped open and subsequently managed 10 retail stores and 18 service centers. We helped an average of 100+ hearing impaired people a month hear better. It was a truly rewarding experience. The industry is unique. You either really enjoy working with the hearing impaired or you don't. I found it very rewarding.

After that, I was asked to join the Home Office of the company and traveled throughout the USA, doing sales, business consulting, and dispenser training.

This career spanned almost 20 years, during which time I had the privilege of working with some of the finest people in the industry, many of whom are still there today. You know who you are.

A Brief History of Hearing Aids

Every publication I have read says that the first hearing aid was created sometime in the 17th century. Major progress toward 'modern' hearing aids did not really occur until after the creation of the telephone and the microphone, in the 1870s and 1880s. Telephone technology provided, for the first time, the ability to alter loudness, frequency, and distortion of sound.

The first electric hearing aid was developed in1898 by Miller Reese Hutchinson and was called the Akouphone. One of the first major manufacturers of electronically amplified hearing aids was the Siemens Company. They started manufacturing hearing aids in 1913. They still manufacture quality hearing aids today, over 100 years later. Those first hearing aids were similar in size to a tall cigar box, and had a speaker that 'somewhat' fit in the ear. Transistor hearing aids appeared in 1948, developed by Bell Laboratories thus continuing the movement toward smaller, more efficient instruments.

While there were certainly improvements in technology over the years, digital hearing aids did not become readily available until the late 20th century. The first ones to become commercially available were developed by Nicolet Corporation in 1987. While Nicolet did not remain in business it did start the competition between other companies to invent more effective hearing aids. In 1989 the first behind the ear digital-analog hybrid hearing aids were introduced. My research shows that Resound Corporation was the first to hit the market with these hybrids. The first ALL-digital hearing aid to become widely available to consumers was created by Widex in 1996. Oticon developed one a year earlier than that but it was only available to audiological research centers.

Frankly, digital hearing aids have revolutionized the industry. They enabled dispensers to adjust hearing aids electronically, thus giving them the ability to 'fine tune' amplification to each patient's individual loss.

One of the true pioneers in the industry was Ken Dahlberg. An outstanding book on his life, *One Step Forward, The Life of Ken Dahlberg*, was first published in 2008. He is perhaps better known as the founder of Dahlberg Electronics, parent company of Miracle-Ear, still one of the largest marketers of hearing aids in the USA. He founded Dahlberg Electronics in 1948. That history starts on page 113 of the above mentioned book. I had the privilege of working for Ken. He was not only an entrepreneur but also a highly decorated World War II fighter ace. He is credited with the first use of the transistor in a consumer product. Ken passed on October 4, 2011 at the age of 94. The industry lost a giant that day.

"Early Thursday", Ken! RIP.

Let's just say we have come a long way from the days of the ear trumpet.

I could write a complete book on Hearing Loss but for the purpose here I am going to give you an abbreviated version. You can thank me later.

The most recent statistics I can find say that there are over 40 MILLION individuals in the USA with some degree of hearing loss. Sadly, less than 25% of those have purchased hearing aids. One thing is certain; when you have major hearing loss it affects both the quality of your life and your relationships. Both of my parents were hearing impaired. I can certainly attest to that.

Let's look first at what are considered to be the major causes of hearing loss. Obviously, normal aging is the most common cause. Let's face it, as we all get older, many things change, hearing is but one of them. Research says that one out of three; between the age of 65 and 74 have some degree of hearing loss. After age 75, make that one out of two.

So let's briefly cover the other things that we KNOW cause hearing loss.

First, and probably foremost, after aging, is noise. Almost 50% of all carpenters have hearing loss, for example. Certainly many of us who were in the military have a loss, but so do those who worked in such industries as mining and manufacturing. Did you listen to loud music growing up? Add that to the list. Every time a car pulls up next to me with their radio at full volume, so loud that the bass rocks MY car, I want to hand them a business card. They WILL need hearing aids in their lifetime. Are they just too dumb to care?

Next on our list are medications. Antibiotics, chemotherapy drugs, or even aspirin and drugs used to treat ED are known villains. Often times these same drugs also affect balance.

Many serious illnesses have also been linked to hearing loss. Heart disease, high blood pressure, and diabetes appear to be the leaders. Does everyone who has one of these diseases also have hearing loss? Of course not, but many do.

While the list of possible causes is long, several others deserve mention here. Sudden hearing loss, defined as a loss of at least 30 decibels, and usually affecting only one ear; trauma, such as a skull fracture; a punctured eardrum; and finally, infections of the ear; and ear wax – although ear wax usually only "reduces" acuity around 5 decibels.

One of the major problems with hearing loss is that it usually develops over a long period of time. As a result, the person suffering from that loss often thinks that people are merely mumbling, that their spouse simply needs to speak up, that the telephone is simply an inferior device, and that all televisions are not turned up adequately. Sound familiar? Admit it, sure it does.

Most hearing loss occurs in the high frequencies and those frequencies are found in children's and most female voices. Those are the frequencies where we find the consonants such as S, P, TH and CH, and SH. If you have hearing loss, you probably may have trouble telling the difference between peace and peach, or cheese and chief.

Most individuals with a hearing loss have varying degrees of difficulty hearing in noisy environments, trouble following more than one conversation at a time, misunderstanding and responding inappropriately, complain that the TV is not loud enough, ask people to repeat themselves, and often have tinnitus (those ringing, roaring, or hissing sounds).

Most textbooks categorize hearing loss into one of four levels and most people seem to progress through these levels. The levels are mild, moderate, severe, and profound.

MILD

With only a mild loss, you probably do fine with one on one conversation unless there is a lot of background noise. If there is, you usually have some trouble understanding some of the words. Usually you blame that on the fact that the person you are talking to simply is not talking loud enough, or that they mumble.

MODERATE

When your hearing loss progresses to the moderate level, you may find yourself asking people to repeat themselves, both face to face and on the telephone.

SEVERE

A severe hearing loss makes it almost impossible to understand a normal conversation. Frustration is often seen here. Many times that escalates to anger or the appearance of anger.

PROFOUND

Profound hearing loss is often referred to as a loss where the person "can't hear thunder". That may be an exaggeration but the person really cannot hear others speaking unless they almost shout. The ability to understand speech is severely limited. At this stage of loss, isolation is often seen. The hearing impaired person chooses not to go to social activities because of their inability to hear well enough to participate in them. Unfortunately, those individuals with a profound loss usually do not benefit from hearing aids as much as those with a lesser degree of loss. We often say they have waited too long to get help.

Treatment for Hearing Loss

In some cases treatment other than a hearing aid is possible. Obviously, that depends upon the type of hearing loss as well as the source. Surgery can often reverse a loss if it is caused by Otosclerosis, a disease primarily of the bones of the middle ear, scar tissue, and sometimes, infection. Meniere's disease, a disease which can include vertigo, hearing loss, and tinnitus (a ringing, roaring, or buzzing in the ears) is sometimes treatable with a combination of medication and/or diet changes.

If none of these options are appropriate, the only avenue usually left to the hearing impaired person is to obtain and use hearing aids. Unfortunately, only about one in four hearing impaired individuals has chosen to do that.

In addition to hearing aids, there are several things family and friends can do to help the hearing impaired person. First, **make sure you are in the same room**, that you have their attention, that they can see your lips, and that you speak clearly without shouting. Common sense, for sure, but often overlooked by many. Even a person with excellent hearing cannot always hear someone from two or three rooms away with the TV or radio on in the background.

What Hearing Aids Are - And What They Are Not

Be very clear about one thing. Hearing aids do not 'restore' hearing. Technology has come light years since the late 80s, but even today hearing aids are not perfect. Don't let anyone tell you otherwise. If they do, they are not the person you should be working with. I've actually heard dispensers say, "You'll hear like you did when you were 20". That simply isn't usually the case.

What they can do is substantially improve your ability to hear, more importantly, understand, in a vast number of different environments. Will there be situations in your everyday life where they won't help as much as you would like them to? Of course there will be.

One of the most common situations where someone wearing hearing aids almost always has a problem is understanding in a noisy environment where the ambient background noise, music, other conversations, dishes, etc., is simply louder than normal conversation. Most noise, regardless of its source, is found in the lower frequencies, overriding if you will the higher frequencies where most speech sounds are heard.

Digital hearing aids that have been properly programmed have substantially eased this problem. Substantially. But they have not entirely eliminated it. Most hearing impaired individuals rapidly learn what restaurants to avoid because of this issue and also learn other ways to adapt to get the most benefit from their hearing aids. Additional guidance is always provided on this by their dispenser. Take notes.

The bottom line is this. Hearing aids, properly programmed, offer major improvement in the area of understanding in most situations. While they are not a be-all cure-all they do offer the hearing impaired the best chance for "quality of life improvement". and improved relationships with family and friends. The fact that most hearing aids today are small enough to be almost invisible has taken that excuse away. Gone are the days when vanity often overruled everything else. That's absolutely a good thing.

How Hearing Aids Work

I'm sure that most everyone reading this book knows basically how hearing aids work so I won't spend a lot time on the subject, but just in case you don't know, here goes.

The principle behind hearing aids is really quite simple. They make conversation easier to understand by making it louder, by frequency, while, at the same time, electronically reducing background noise.

They do that through the use of several components. The basic components of every hearing aid are the microphone that picks up the sound waves and converts them into electricity so they can be digitized, and the digital processor/amplifier that takes the electrical signals sent by the microphone and changes them into digital signals. Enhancements to the original sound, such as frequency amplification, noise and wind reduction, and feedback cancellation happen here. And finally, the signal is then converted back into sound waves by the receiver and sent to the brain, via the middle and inner ear.

Some hearing aids today still have a volume control, but most adjust the volume automatically as you move from one listening environment to the next.

Finally, power to the hearing aid is provided by a small battery. Most hearing aids use a zinc-air battery, which is not 'activated' until you remove a clearly marked paper tab. Batteries last anywhere from 3-5 days up to perhaps 2 weeks, depending primarily upon the functions being performed by the hearing aid and the number of hours per day that they are used. Replacement batteries cost $1.00 each or less. It is always a good idea to buy batteries from someone who sells them frequently to ensure that you are getting fresh ones. Battery 'shelf life' varies, but is usually at least a year. I recommend that you buy your batteries from your dispenser. Most offer battery 'clubs' which reduce the individual cost. Hearing aid dispensers usually have the freshest batteries. Buying batteries by mail is usually not the best idea, freshness wise. As with most things, you really do get what you pay for. I have found a lot of individuals, too many, actually, are obsessed with battery life. Many can't understand why a hearing aid battery does not last as long as a watch battery. The answer is simple. A LOT more is going on within the hearing aid circuit than with your watch. Batteries last as long as they do. Many improvements in battery life have been made over the years. Please consider the cost of batteries just one of the prices you pay to hear better.

Hearing aids vary in price, size, features, and how they fit into the ears.

CIC

The smallest of all hearing aids is the 'completely in the canal' hearing aid (CIC, for short). It is the least visible hearing aid made. It picks up the least amount of wind noise, and it uses the smallest battery and with that usually comes the shortest battery life and one that can also be difficult to install and remove for anyone with dexterity problems. It fits totally inside your ear canal. The CICs normally are too small for either a volume control or directional microphones and are usually more susceptible to becoming plugged with ear wax. Additionally, they may not be able to adequately help someone with a loss that is greater than mild to moderate. Regardless of what you have heard, size does matter to most. Everyone who buys a hearing aid wants it to be invisible, while at the same time giving them the help they need in 100% of the daily situations they experience. We used to say that hearing loss is far more visible than any hearing aid but vanity still rules. Don't let anyone kid you about that. You may personally be a candidate for this size hearing aid, or not. Your dispenser is best qualified to help you with that decision.

ITC

The next size up is the 'in the canal' hearing aid (ITC). Like the CIC, it is custom molded (using an actual impression of the ear canal made out of silicone) but it fits only partly into the ear canal.

The canal hearing aid is less visible than larger sizes but it certainly does have more visibility than the CIC. While it accommodates features that the CIC does not, it may still be difficult to adjust, insert, and remove, because of size. It is also more susceptible to earwax clogging.

ITE

The 'in the ear' (ITE) hearing aid is also custom made, and usually available in two styles. The first style fills most of the bowl of the outer ear and is called a full shell ITE. The other style only fills the lower part of the bowl of the outer ear and is call a half shell ITE. Both are capable of offering more power than either the CIC or the ITC. Both are large enough for a volume control as well as directional microphones, and, based upon their size, are easier for most people to adjust. They are also easier to insert and remove, and use a larger battery (think easier to change and longer life). The downside to this size is they may pick up more wind noise than smaller models and they are more visible.

BTE

The 'behind the ear' (BTE) hearing aids hook over the top of your ears and rest behind them. I'm sure you have noticed that I refer to hearing aids, plural. As with vision, most people with hearing loss normally have a similar loss in each ear. One hearing aid only helps one ear. If you are tempted to only buy one which I totally and completely recommend AGAINST, ask yourself which ear you don't want to hear well with. Those individuals who only buy one hearing aid are seldom satisfied. One of the reasons for this is that the ear they did not buy a hearing aid for continues to hear all the background noise, but does not hear the high frequencies. The BTE hearing aids are appropriate for anyone, of any age, and with almost any degree of hearing loss. They are, however, the largest and most visible of all hearing aids.

RIC

Fairly new to the market is the 'receiver in the canal' (RIC) hearing aid, also called the receiver in the ear. This is my personal favorite. You see more and more of these. While they are worn behind the ear, they are much smaller and far less visible than the traditional BTE. They give excellent sound reproduction. One variation of this type of hearing aid is the open fit model. The open fit hearing aid keeps the ear canal 'open' more than any other model. This allows for most low frequency sounds to enter the ear naturally and for high frequency sounds, normally described as those sounds that are over 1000 Hertz, to receive the most amplification.

Who Should Buy Them? - The Ideal Candidate

It would be wonderful if everyone was a perfect candidate for hearing aids. That's just not the case. I'll cover those that I think should not buy them in the next chapter. Here we will concentrate on those who I feel are ideal candidates.

First, the younger a person is when they accept their hearing loss and decide to seek help, the better.

Second, the person who is still active socially will obviously benefit more from hearing aids than the person who never leaves their home. I remember my mother was an avid bridge player. Prior to getting hearing aids she had basically quit playing. After she got them, she was playing twice a week again. She could hear the bid again. Anyone who has ever worked in this industry has many similar stories similar to this and frankly, that's one of the intangible benefits to a career in the industry.

Third, it does take a degree of patience to adjust to hearing aids. If you are hearing impaired, that hearing loss probably did not happen overnight. Likewise, learning to hear with hearing aids gets easier over time, and it does take some time. Most dispensers recommend a "get used to them" program that lasts anywhere from 30 to 90 days. That time frame has been reduced as a result of digital hearing aids but it has not been totally eliminated. During that time you will meet with your dispenser several times to make sure you are receiving maximum benefit from your purchase. He or she normally has equipment to measure the performance of the hearing aids while they are in your ears. They may reprogram them during those meetings. Occasionally, a 'fit' problem will need to be corrected. This is usually only true with aids other than the RICs.

Fourth, and in my opinion the most important, is YOUR desire and commitment to hear well. The more you WANT to hear better, the more effort you will put into achieving that goal and the more that same effort will pay off for you. Motivated users ALWAYS do better than those who have purchased hearing aids for the wrong reasons, which I will cover in the next chapter.

Who Should Probably Not Buy Them?

At first glance, a person would think that everyone who has hearing loss should just rush out and buy hearing aids. If only it were that simple. It's not. There are actually people who probably should not buy hearing aids. Not a huge group of them, but certainly some. Here are several reasons why I feel it may be better not to buy them.

First, buying them only to get a family member or your spouse 'off your back'. That's probably the absolute worst reason of all to buy hearing aids. The thought process is simple. My wife thinks I need hearing aids. While I have been shown that I do have hearing loss, and that loss would perhaps benefit from hearing aids, I simply do not want to buy them, much less wear them. Period. My wife can speak up and she can get used to the fact that I like the TV louder than she does. So there. You probably even know somebody like that. Perhaps it's even YOU.

Second, you have basically no social life. You live alone. You don't go to church or even go out for that matter. Who cares if you have the TV a 'little' louder these days, right? This is amplified if you have no adult children. However, I have seen people like this who have purchased hearing aids and who actually developed a new, active, social life as a result. Who would have thought? Hearing aids also provide a safety element in cases like this. Hearing the fire alarm is always a good thing, as is hearing the telephone ring.

Third, you have very limited dexterity and no one to help you put them in and take them off, let alone change the batteries. Frankly, that's probably the first really valid reason so far! And even that one has solutions.

Fourth, like a lack of dexterity, a lack of vision can also become a real problem if you don't have anybody to help you, such as a spouse.

Does 'Brand' Matter?

During my tenure in the industry, I only worked with one company. Perhaps you may have guessed which one by now. As a result, I'm only thoroughly familiar with the hearing aids that company sells. However, there are a number of other reliable hearing aid manufactures in the market place today. As long as you purchase hearing aids made by one of them you will be assured of quality, good service, and hearing aids that will give you years of service. Here is a list of companies that I think are in that category. PLEASE do not view this list as the only good companies out there because it is not intended to be. At last count, there were about 40 companies manufacturing hearing aids. All the companies I have listed below have been in business for a long time.

I have listed them in alphabetical order to preclude any bias on my part. Please don't stop here. Do some homework.

Also remember that both Beltone and Miracle-Ear have their own brands.

Beltone manufactures its own hearing aids. Great Nordic Store, Copenhagen, owns both Beltone and Resound.

The hearing aids Miracle-Ear sells are manufactured for them by a dedicated, state of the art, Siemens' manufacturing facility.

Beltone
GNResound
Miracle-Ear
Oticon
Phonak/Unitron
Rexton
Siemens
Starkey
Widex

How Much Technology Do You Really Need?

This is really a fairly easy question to answer based upon your individual situation.

Almost all quality hearing aids manufactured today use digital technology. The decisions you need to make are thus limited. Some decisions that remain are how many channels you need. More channels simply mean more frequency points that a dispenser can adjust. An 8 channel system means that the dispenser can 'address' and adjust 8 frequencies. A 16 channel system doubles that number. Personally, I think that anything beyond 16 channels borders on overkill, and anything below 8 is probably not enough.

Many hearing aids today offer a remote control, allowing you to adjust various things about the hearing aids without touching or removing them, volume, listening program, etc. When remote controls were first introduced they were very popula, the latest whistle and bell, if you like. Do you need a remote control? If you are a high tech individual who likes to have the latest gadget, the answer is probably yes, without question. Most hearing aids work just fine without a remote control.

Many other features, such as dual microphones, are popular. Dual mics make sense in many listening situations. Your dispenser can explain all the available options to you so you can decide which ones you need as opposed to which ones might be nice. Everyone has different demands of their hearing aids. And everyone has different financial ability. I'm not in favor or simply paying more because you can. Sure, you can do that, but I think everyone should weigh the benefits of hearing aids against the cost.

What I will say, without reservation, is this. DO NOT buy any hearing aid that does not use digital technology. Yes, you will pay more for digital technology, but it's like flying in a plane with propellers versus jets. Digital technology has truly revolutionized the industry. Take advantage of that.

Where to Buy Them and Why

Hearing aids are sold many places. Many otolaryngologists have an audiologist on staff. Many audiologists also sell hearing aids in their private practices. Licensed hearing aid dispensers are perhaps the most prevalent source of hearing aids.

So where should YOU buy yours? Frankly, that's not a one size fits all question.

As with most everything any of us buy, price determines a number of things. With the purchase of a hearing aid, there are many factors that go into determining price. Buying the lowest priced hearing aid is seldom the best answer for a number of reasons. First, all hearing aids take time to get used to. If you buy a hearing aid from a Big Box store the time their dispenser has available to help you after the sale could be limited. One of the biggest complaints I hear is that, while their prices are usually the lowest, their customers are frequently not happy with the service they get after the sale. Many of those customers go to another dispenser or an audiologist to seek help. However it is important to remember that hearing aids today require less 'adjustments' then those in the past.

My own otolaryngologist, a friend of mine, has an audiologist on his staff. His office is relatively close to a Big Box store with a hearing aid department. He recently told me they see someone almost every week that purchased their hearing aids from a Big Box store and haven't been satisfied with the service they received after the sale. Am I saying don't buy a hearing aid from a Big Box store? Absolutely not. A number of current dispensers for one such store have actually worked with and for me in the past and I've personally trained several others who work there. Big box stores have some really good dispensers, if I do say so myself. They sell quality products for less than most of their competition. What I am saying is that with hearing aids, perhaps more so than most other products, initial cost should not be the only factor that you look at when you are dealing with hearing loss. If you simply can't get the service you need one of two things will happen. First, you will simply give up and quit wearing the hearing aids. That happens in far too many cases. We call those the in the drawer model. Second, you will find someone else and buy another pair of hearing aids for more than you originally spent on the first ones. So was the low price you originally paid really a bargain? You know the answer to that one as well as I do.

The VA and the Big Box stores currently account for 40% of all hearing aids sold in the U.S. That's a LOT of hearing aids. I'll discuss the VA later in this book.

Audiologists are highly trained to identify and treat hearing and speech problems, including hearing loss. However their education is limited when it comes to the actual dispensing of hearing aids and most of them will be the first to admit that.

Hearing aid dispensers are licensed and regulated by most, if not all, states. The requirements to obtain a license are stringent and there is an annual continuing educational requirement as well. Hearing aid dispensers can be broken down into two general categories, those that carry only one brand, such as dealers for Beltone or Miracle-Ear, and those that carry a broad number of brands. I've never really understood the need to offer every brand on the market. Every brand that I know about is available with pretty much the same technology and usually in the same sizes. From a personal point of view, were I to need hearing aids, which, so far, I do not (although my wife might not agree!). I would opt to go with a hearing aid dispenser. Perhaps that's because I once was one, but more so because I have worked with so many good ones over the years. They will take the time they need to help you adjust to yours. And you will find that you really won't pay substantially more than you could have paid elsewhere.

Why Mail Order Hearing Aids Are Usually a Mistake

You can't pick up a Sunday newspaper without finding at least one ad for hearing aids. The companies offering them usually skirt the FDA regulations by calling them something other than a hearing aid. Listening device is a frequently used term in the ads. The low price should be a dead giveaway to the fact that they won't provide the kind of help most people need. If you fall for the hype, you will usually be unable to get any service locally. Most reputable dispensers won't touch them. Bottom line, if you need help with your hearing the Sunday newspaper is probably not the best place to start. One size absolutely does not fit all when it comes to a hearing aid. Save your time and money.

There are also a couple of companies out there that actually sell a somewhat better product by mail. Legally, there are a number of states that they can't even ship into but that doesn't seem to stop them.

Hearing loss is too important to treat this way. Do it right. You will be glad you did.

What to Look For In A Dispenser and Why

OK, you have decided that it's time to get serious about your hearing loss and take some action. Where should you start? One place a person can start is with a visit to their ear doctor to rule out any medical problems that might preclude them from benefiting from hearing aids. However, the FDA does allow a person to sign a medical waiver indicating that they have been advised to see a medical professional prior to buying hearing aids. Frankly, dispersers and audiologists are trained to spot medical problems regarding your ears and your hearing. When they do spot such a problem, they are required, by law, to refer you to a doctor. I know of no one who would not do that. I'm not suggesting you sign the waiver, just making you aware of the fact that you can do that.

Regardless, the first step in the process is often to have your hearing and understanding evaluated. Most dispensers will do this for you at no charge with the hope that you will buy hearing aids from them. Most audiologists will charge for this service. The evaluation itself will consist of several parts. First, they will conduct what is called a pure tone test testing your ability to hear tones over a frequency range of between usually 500 Hertz and 8000 Hertz. Hertz. Named after **Heinrich Rudolf Hertz** (German: [hɛʁts]; 22 February 1857 – 1 January 1894).

The tones will either be continuous or intermittent. You will be instructed to either raise your hand or push a button every time you hear one. Every frequency will normally be tested at least twice. During your test you will most likely wear headphones, which were apparently not designed to be comfortable, because they seldom are! The person conducting the test will record your responses on a form called an Audiogram, which they will explain to you after they have completed your entire evaluation. There will also be one or more additional tests conducted to determine your speech threshold, and your level of understanding. Normally, a thorough evaluation takes between 45 and 75 minutes.

Sorry, I digressed. What to look for in a dispenser was the topic. First look for someone who you feel listens to you. If they are not asking you questions about the situations where you are having problems and how those situations are affecting your daily life, perhaps they are not the person you should be working with.

Second, go with your gut feeling, either you basically like the dispenser or you don't. Only work with those you like. You will be spending a fair amount of time with them over the first few months after you buy hearing aids. Do they have the patience you are seeking? Are they empathetic? Do you feel they are knowledgeable? It's absolutely OK to ask them about their experience. How long have they been dispensing? Are they licensed to dispense in your state? How long have they been licensed? What hours are they available? Can you reach them after normal business hours or on weekends if you need to? These are the questions I'd personally want answers to before I would even consider buying hearing aids for anyone. You may even have additional ones. Your success with hearing aids depends on two things, your commitment, and their expertise. One without the other will not result in success.

How Much Do You Really Need To Spend?

This may well be the most difficult question for me to answer. I remember I used to ask people that I tested if they would wear hearing aids if they were free. Surprisingly, not everyone answered yes to that question. Cost is seldom the real reason a person does not get the help they need for their hearing loss. Fact.

So I am going to give you a range, based upon prices today. Remember, most hearing losses benefit from two hearing aids, so you need to take these prices and double them.

I would be concerned with any digital hearing aid that I was offered that sold for less than $1250 each. On the other end of the spectrum, it's possible to pay $3000 or more for a hearing aid. As a general rule, I would look to pay something in the range of $2500 to $5000 for a PAIR of quality hearing aids.

How long do hearing aids last, and will I need to replace them? Those are totally appropriate and frequently asked questions. How long will a hearing aid last? I have seen hearing aids that were still working well after 25 years. Certainly a number more that were over 10 years old. Rule of thumb, I think it's reasonable to expect a hearing aid to last at least 10 years.

Will you need to replace them? Need is probably the key word here. With programmable digital hearing aids, you may not have a need to replace them unless your hearing loss worsens to the point where the original hearing aids can no longer adequately correct the problem. Will technology continue to improve as the years go by? Of course it will. Might you want to get new technology at some point in time? Sure you might. Only you can be the judge of that. When I first started fitting hearing aids, they were all analog. Those hearing aids were manufactured to correct the loss found during the hearing evaluation. We would send a copy of the audiogram and the speech testing to the manufacturer, and they would make hearing aids designed to correct THAT loss. As the patient's loss became worse over time, we often had to start over with new hearing aids because the original set simply no longer offered the help they needed. Back then, it was certainly not uncommon to replace hearing aids every 3-5 years. With today's technology, that is usually not necessary.

Does Medicare Pay For Hearing Aids?

I am told that before I started dispensing hearing aids Medicare did pay for them. Unfortunately, that is no longer the case. Apparently, everyone who even remotely needed hearing aids got them back then. Hey, they were free. What can I say? That used to be the case with the motorized scooters so many people have. I think the Scooter Store debacle has somewhat reduced that.

Ironically, Medicaid does still pay for them. Go figure. However, the aids that are provided to Medicaid patients are certainly not top of the line in most cases. I don't think I have ever met a Medicaid patient who was truly happy with their hearing aids.

Some insurance companies have hearing aid benefits. A number of other groups, such as the NRA, AARP, and AMAC have providers who will offer discounts. If price is a major issue to you, shop around. While the discounts are usually never substantial they do offer some help.

What's More Important Than Cost?

What could possibly be more important than cost? Simply this. Do the hearing aids offer me the help I need to hear better in the majority of situations that are important to me? If the hearing aids cost $1000 each and you can't hear any better than you did before you got them, they were not a bargain.

Likewise, if the hearing aids cost $3000 each and they allow you to hear much better all of the time, they probably were a bargain.

Bottom line, the most important thing about hearing aids is not so much their cost but their ability to give you an improved quality of life through the better hearing that you seek. That is priceless to most. Remember, I have been in the trenches in this industry. I've seen lives CHANGED as a result of hearing aids. I've seen marriages saved, families reunited, happiness restored, and lives lengthened. I've seen it all or at least a lot of it. Do I think hearing aids are worth every dime you pay for them? You bet I do. And you will too if you take advantage of the help that is out there today.

Is It Difficult To Get Used To Hearing Aids?

With the digital technology found pretty much throughout the industry today, it's easier to get used to hearing aids now than it has ever been in the past. Two major problems with hearing aids in the past, especially when they were analog, were a plugged up feeling and an inability to hear well in noise.. Analog hearing aids were only adjustable with trim pots (formally called potentiometers) that were adjusted by the dispenser with a screw driver, and with venting-modifying the shell of the hearing aid to allow for more natural reception of the low frequencies which was frequently accomplished with a Dremel drill. Both had limitations. Today, almost all hearing aids are 100% digital and as such, programmable by frequency.

In years past we used to tell people to get used to their new hearing aids by following a wearing schedule, i.e., wear them 2 hours the first day, four hours the second, etc., until they were comfortable wearing them from the time they got up until the time they went to bed.

Today we normally tell a new user to just put them in and wear them. That's appropriate unless the person is a highly nervous individual and in those cases we still discuss an initial wearing schedule. Remember, you did not come by your hearing loss overnight. Don't expect to be able to simply put new hearing aids in and hear as well as you are going to. Your hearing acuity will usually improve over time and that time may well be up to 90 days. Again, your commitment to hearing better is a prime factor.

Managing Expectations

In that same regard, let's talk a little bit about expectations. Many new users get discouraged because they still can't hear the way they think they should in ALL situations. Even a person with no hearing loss does not hear perfectly in every situation. The objective of hearing aids is to help you hear and, more importantly, understand, better in "most" situations. If, for example, you go into a really noisy environment, such as a crowded restaurant, there will still be parts of conversations that you may miss. We have come light years with digital technology, and a properly programmed digital instrument WILL enable you to hear better in almost all situations. Such things as where you sit make a difference. Sitting with your back to as much of the noise as you can certainly helps. Being able to see the person you are talking to helps. Everyone tends to do some lip reading, intentionally or not. The point I want to make is simply this, maintain your commitment to hearing and understanding better. Over time you will see improvements. Don't expect them all to happen on day one. They won't.

I'm A Veteran - Should I See the VA?

I am a veteran. If you are too, and suspect you have a hearing loss (or know that you do), you will probably consider seeing the VA about that.

Some questions, however, are in order.

First, are you currently eligible for VA benefits and/or already receiving them or can you enroll to obtain them? When I left the military I did not enroll in that program.

Second, do you live close enough to a VA facility to make it convenient for you to get your hearing aids there and to get them serviced there?

Third, are you currently able to drive or do you have someone who can drive you there? Do you see that changing soon?

So the question comes down to this. Can I get hearing aids from the VA?

I have taken the liberty of copying the following from this source about eligibility for hearing aids from the VA.
http://www.visn2.va.gov/dt/audiologyfaqs.asp#q1

"It is National VA Policy that hearing aids are furnished to eligible veterans in accordance with the restrictions defined in VA Directive 2002-039 released July 5, 2002. Briefly, the Directive explains that eligibility for hearing aids is currently limited to veterans with a documented service connected hearing loss, veterans receiving a disability rating of 10% or more – for a condition other than hearing loss, and some veterans with very special needs.

With the exception of veterans with documented service connection for hearing loss, an eligible veteran must be currently enrolled in and receiving healthcare from a VISN 2 VA Medical Center or Outpatient Clinic.

Hearing aids are not customarily provided to non-service connected veterans. However, if there is a medical reason, a VA Physician can refer a non-service connected veteran for a hearing evaluation.

If you are not certain about your eligibility status, check the blue pages of your local phone directory for the number of your local Veterans Benefits counselor or call your nearest VA and ask for the Veterans Service Center.

We all know that the VA is not long on funds and since 9/11 there have been a lot of demands for those funds. There have also been a lot of changes within the VA system as it pertains to hearing aids in the last 7-10 years. More of the major manufacturers have taken an interest in this aspect of the industry and the VA has negotiated contracts with several of them to provide the best products they manufacture. The contract period is now 5 years with product updates every 6 months. The current (2015) suppliers are GNResound, Starkey, Siemens, Phonak/Unitron, Oticon, and Widex.

One thing that has not changed is the amount of time it may take a veteran to be initially seen by the VA for hearing loss. And the product they receive will be the one their audiologist happens to like best, unless there is a strong reason to request something specific.

The hearing aids dispensed by the VA today are state of the art. I have always found the people who dispense hearing aids within the VA system to be both knowledgeable and professional.

If you are a veteran, currently receiving VA benefits or can become eligible for them, meet the requirements above, and their location is convenient for you, by all means explore what they have to offer. The VA also provides hearing aid batteries if you obtain hearing aids through them.

I have personally fit a lot of veterans who decided not to go the VA route for a variety of reasons or who went to them initially and sought out more help after that. Some simply lived too far from a VA Clinic to make it convenient for them to use the VA. Just like any one dispenser, the VA may or may not be right for you. Only you can make that call.

Warranties and Return Policies

I don't know of any hearing aid manufactured that does not automatically come with at least a one year warranty. What does that warranty cover? It covers the hearing aid if it quits working and the problem cannot be fixed in the dispenser's office. Many hearing aids come with longer warranties – some up to three years in length. My own thoughts on warranties is simple; if a hearing aid is going to fail electronically, it will most likely do that in the first year, frankly, usually within the first month or so. And that simply does not happen very often. Quality control in the manufacturing process of hearing aids is extensive. So is a warranty longer than a year really a big deal? Probably not. Another provision often found is what is called a loss and damage warranty. It covers your hearing aids if you lose one or both of them, or if the dog (or cat) eats them.

NOTE: The loss and damage provision of most warranties is only good one time per aid. Don't laugh. I have actually seen that happen. I personally fit a lady in Mesa AZ who had two miniature French poodles. They ate her new hearing aids. All she found in the back yard was a short piece of small copper wire (less than an inch long) and one battery. Talk about expensive dog food. Fortunately she had loss and damage coverage and we made her a new pair of hearing aids at no cost. When she first called me, she had forgotten that she had that coverage. She was in tears. We always warn new users to keep their hearing aids out of reach of pets. For a reason.

Let's talk about return policies. Some dispensers I have met tend to sell what I call trials. "Try these and if you don't like them give them back." This sets up a failure scenario. A person buys new hearing aids; they "try" them for a week or so, don't seem to be adjusting to them as well as they had hoped, so they just give them back. That's a disservice to them. It is, however, part of the industry. Every state dictates that the buyer of hearing aids be given a refund, sometimes less a fitting fee, if they ask for it within a certain time period, usually 30 days. Unfortunately, a lot of new users have not fully adjusted to hearing with hearing aids by then. So when you buy your hearing aids, I suggest that you ask for a 45-60 day 'get used to them' return period. Your dispenser wants to see you do well with your hearing aids. They will work hard to help you do that. The more time you give them, the better the outcome.

Conclusion

OK, there you have it. I hope you have enjoyed reading this Layman's Guide as much as I have truly enjoyed writing it. I have a passion for this industry. Maybe it shows. It was good to me for a lot of years. I can proudly say that I helped a LOT of people to hear and understand better during those years. I hope by writing this that I have at least motivated you to get help for your hearing loss. Life is too precious to waste. No longer does someone with a hearing loss have to be left out of a portion of it.

I don't aspire to become a famous author. What I do aspire to do is help as many people as I can during those years that I have left. If this book has helped you I have achieved that goal.

If it has, I'd be very grateful if you would take just a few minutes to write a short review on Amazon so that this book might help even more people experiencing hearing loss.

Thank you so much.

Thomas Shaw

Resources

For those of you who seek additional information, I have listed several sources. Some of these are textbooks that I have used in my own study of hearing loss.

Just call this section a bonus.

Hearing Instrument Science & Fitting Practices, Robert E. Sandlin

Hearing Instrument Counseling, Max X. Chartrand

Fundamentals of Hearing: An Introduction, William A. Yost

Instrumentation in Audiology and Hearing Science: Theory and Practice, Shlomo Silman and Michele B. Emmer

Fitting and Dispensing Hearing Aids, Brian Taylor and H. Gustav Mueller

Introduction To Sound: Acoustics for the Hearing and Speech Sciences, Charles E. Speaks.

Hearing Aid Handbook, Jeffrey J. DiGiovanni

Electronics and Instrumentation for Audiologists, Paul J. Moser

Handbook of Signal Processing in Acoustics, (2 Volume Set), David Havelock and Sonoko Kuwano

Foundations of Aural Rehabilitation: Children, Adults, and Their Family Members, Nancy Tye-Murray

Digital Hearing Aids, Arthur Schaub

www.ingramcontent.com/pod-product-compliance
Lightning Source LLC
Chambersburg PA
CBHW061935280526
45787CB00004B/1611